Ketogenic Diet

The Ultimate Guide For Rapid Weight Loss, Boost Your Energy And Heal Your Body

(How You Can Lose Weight The Easy Way Through A Keto Diet)

Larry Doyle

TABLE OF CONTENTS

Ketogenic Bolognese Sauce 1

Mediterranean Tuna Keto Pizza 4

Trout 6

Gaucho Keto Burger 8

Salmon In A Zucchini Bed 10

Burgers Keto Pesto 12

Keto Pesto 13

Chicken And Cauliflower Casserole With Keto Pesto 15

Chicken Roulade With Pesto 17

Almond Cod With Braised Tomatoes 20

Fillet Of Beef With Brussels Sprouts 22

Pollock In A Coconut-Lime Coating On Spinach 24

Chicken On A Feta-Spinach Bed 26

Bacon And Pinach Frittata 27

Pumpkin Fries 30

Chicken And Cabbage Rolls With Sesame Soy Dip 32

Turkey Breast With Cheese Sauce 35

Baked Mini Peppers 37
Tex Mex Casserole 39
Baked Celery Root With Gorgonzola 41
Bacon Cheeseburger Wraps 43
Fish Casserole With Mushrooms And French Mustard 45
Keto Quiche With Bacon And Spinach 48
Marinated Cold Broccoli Salad With Bacon 50
Gingerbread Bombs 52
Zucchini Brownies 54
Chia Seed Pudding With Strawberries 57
Lamb Barbacoa 59
Pork Chile Verde 61
Ham Soup 63
Minced Pork Zucchini Lasagna 65
Beef Dijon 67
Cabbage & Corned Beef 70
Chipotle Barbacoa 72
Corned Beef Cabbage Rolls 74
Cube Steak 77
Ragu 79
Rope Vieja 81
Spinach Soup 83

- Mashed Cauliflower With Herbs 84
- Kale Quiche 85
- Sardine Pate 87
- Spare Ribs 88
- Pork Shoulder 90
- Lamb Chops 92
- Rosemary Leg Of Lamb 94
- Creamy Chicken Thighs 95
- Peppered Steak 97
- Rabbit Stew 99
- Duck Breast 100
- Jerk Chicken 101
- Bbq Beef Short Ribs 102
- Spiced Beef 103
- Green Peas Chowder 105
- Chorizo Soup 106
- Spicy Wings With Mint Sauce 107
- Cacciatore Olive Chicken 110
- Duck And Vegetable Stew 111
- Mushroom Cream Goose Curry 112
- Colombian Chicken 114
- Chicken Curry 115

Ketogenic Bolognese Sauce

Ingredients:

- 1/2 teaspoon stevia powder
- 2 tablespoons of double cream
- 2 tablespoon butter
- 2 bay leaf
- 1 tablespoon parsley (fresh)
- 1 tablespoon oregano (fresh)
- 1 tablespoon thyme (fresh)
- 1/2 teaspoon cinnamon (ground)
- 1/2 teaspoon salt
- 1/2 teaspoon pepper
- 10g coconut oil
- 90g breakfast bacon
- 80 g fresh onion
- g garlic

- 290g ground beef
- 250g bratwurst (coarse)
- 290g strained tomatoes
- 250g pizza tomatoes
- 250 ml vegetable stock

Preparation:

1. First, peel the fresh onion and garlic, chop them finely and fry them in a pan with a little coconut oil.
2. Then the bacon must be cut into small pieces and then briefly browned.
3. In the next step, press the sausage meat out of the skin and put it in the pan at the same time as the minced meat.
4. To season the Bolognese sauce, add the spices, stevia extract, salt and pepper.

5. Mix the whole thing together well and let it simmer on the stove for 35 minutes on low heat.
6. Then the tomato sauce, the pizza tomatoes and the broth must be stirred in. Simmer this again for about 35 minutes.
7. At the end remove the bay leaf, stir in the double cream and butter and season to taste.

Mediterranean Tuna Keto Pizza

Ingredients:

- 90g bacon
- 4 0g paprika
- 4 0g fresh onion
- 250 chicory
- 35 0g tuna (in oil)
- 2 fresh egg
- 4 0g cheddar (grated)

Preparation:

1. First, preheat the oven to 2 60 ° C fan-assisted air.
2. Drain the tuna and mix with the fresh egg to a smooth mass.

3. Now cut the fresh onion , bacon and vegetables and fry them in the pan for about 10 minutes.

4. Now the tuna and fresh egg mixture has to be spread out on a tray and then the bacon and vegetables sprinkled on the pizza base .

5. Finally, cover with the cheese and bake in the oven for about 35 minutes.

Trout

Ingredients:

- 2 teaspoon salt
- 4 sprigs of thyme (fresh)
- 2 sprigs of rosemary
- 6 30g trout
- 25ml MCT oil [8]

Preparation:

1. First preheat the oven (setting: grill) to 2 60 ° C.
2. Wash the trout thoroughly under running water, pat dry with kitchen towels and then season with salt.
3. Cut deeply into the trout three times on both sides, place in a deep pan and fill with thyme and rosemary.

4. The trout must then be coated with the MCT oil and put in the oven.
5. After 35 minutes, check the cooking level and, if necessary, increase the temperature to 2 80 ° C.
6. After another 6 -8 minutes, take the fish out of the oven.

Gaucho Keto Burger

Ingredients:

Patties
- 1 teaspoon salt
- Fresh eggs and lettuce
- 2 fried fresh eggs
- 90g leaf lettuce
- 250g ground beef
- 250g Bratwurs tbrät
- 35 g shallots (chopped)
- 2 clove of garlic
- 2 pinch of black pepper
- Pesto
- 80 ml Burger pesto

Preparation:

1. To prepare the patties, combine all the patty ingredients and shape into small circles by hand.
2. Cook the patties on a grill or pan for 35 to 35 minutes.
3. To prepare the other parts of the burger, the fried fresh eggs must be fried in a greased frying pan.
4. Finally, place the patties on lettuce leaves, place the fried fresh egg on the meat and pour the burger pesto over it.
5. The gaucho keto burger is ready .

Salmon In A Zucchini Bed

Ingredients:

- 4 0g fresh onion (red)
- 2 tablespoon olive oil
- 2 clove of garlic
- Thyme (dried)
- Dill (dried)
- Rosemary (fresh)
- 2 salmon fillets
- 2 fresh lemon
- 2 zucchini
- 2 tomatoes
- salt
- pepper

Preparation:

1. Preheat the oven to 350 ºC.
2. In order to prepare the "bed", 2 bowls must be formed from aluminum foil.
3. Now the zucchini and fresh lemon have to be cut into slices and then distributed in the peel.
4. Place the salmon on top of the zucchini and fresh lemon slices.
5. Then chop the tomatoes and chop the fresh onion and garlic.
6. Spread all the ingredients on the salmon.
7. Season to taste with salt and pepper.
8. Put the herbs in the bowls.
9. Close the aluminum foil tightly.
10. Finally bake the finished salmon in the zucchini bed in the oven at 350 ºC for 35 minutes.
11. The salmon in the zucchini bed is now ready to serve.

Burgers Keto Pesto

Ingredients:

- 1 teaspoon salt
- 1 teaspoon pepper (black)
- 2 pinch of chilli flakes
- 8 ml white wine vinegar
- 35 g parsley
- 2 tablespoon oregano (fresh)
- 2 cloves of garlic
- 80 ml olive oil

Preparation:

1. Put all ingredients in a tall container and puree with a hand blender.
2. The burger pesto is ready.

Keto Pesto

Ingredients:

- 1 teaspoon garlic
- 2 teaspoon tomato paste
- 4 basil
- 25g pine nuts
- 30g parmesan
- 8 2ml olive oil

Preparation:

1. First, roast the pine nuts.
2. Then mix all the ingredients in a bowl with a hand blender and slowly add the olive oil.

Chicken And Cauliflower Casserole With Keto Pesto

Ingredients:

- 6 10g tomato
- 4 0g butter (unsalted)
- 2 6g keto pesto (recipe 610)
- 2 teaspoon salt
- 1 teaspoon pepper
- 250 g chicken legs (skinless)
- 2 35 g cheddar
- 250g cream (high fat content)
- 2 90g cauliflower
- 50 g leek

Preparation:

1. First preheat the oven to 2 80 ° C fan oven.
2. The butter must then be heated in a pan and the chicken cut into pieces.
3. Now the chicken has to cook until golden brown in the pan for about 6-8 minutes.
4. Then add the salt and pepper to the chicken.
5. Now the pesto has to be mixed with the cream.
6. Now put the chicken in a baking dish and add the pesto cream.
7. Chop the cauliflower, tomato and leek into pieces and place the vegetables in the baking dish.
8. Cut the cheese into small pieces and sprinkle on top.

9. Bake the casserole for 40 to 45 minutes.

Chicken Roulade With Pesto

Ingredients:

- 1 teaspoon garlic
- 1 teaspoon salt
- 1 teaspoon pepper
- about 2 tablespoons of olive oil
- 2 chicken breast fillets
- 100g Halloumi - grilled cheese [35]
- 250 ml keto pesto (recipe 610)
- 2.10g zest of one fresh lemon

Preparation:

1. First rinse the chicken breast with a little water and then dry it with kitchen paper.
2. Then fillet the chicken breast as thinly as possible and pound it with a meat mallet.
3. Now mix the keto pesto with a tablespoon of olive oil and spread on the chicken breast.
4. Also rub the fresh lemon peel over the chicken.
5. Now cut the halloumi cheese into cube-sized pieces and spread this on the chicken as well.
6. To make roulades, the fillet pieces must now be rolled up and secured with a stick
7. Now preheat the oven to 280 ° C convection.
8. Then fry the roulades in a pan so that all sides turn brown.

9. Finally, the roulades have to be put in the oven for 5-10 minutes and then cooled for about 10 minutes before serving.

Almond Cod With Braised Tomatoes

Ingredients:

- 4 sprigs of thyme
- 30g almond flakes
- 1 fresh lemon
- 400g cherry tomatoes
- 1 bunch of basil
- 2 tablespoon olive oil
- 290 g cod
- 1/2 teaspoon salt
- 1/2 teaspoon pepper

Preparation:

1. Preheat the oven to 250° C with a fan oven.
2. Then heat some olive oil in a pan and fry the fish for 2 minutes on each side.

3. Then season the fish with salt and pepper if you like.
4. Scatter the thyme and flaked almonds over the fish, slice the fresh lemon and place in the pan with the tomatoes.
5. Put the whole pan in the oven until the fish is done and the tomatoes pop open.
6. Before serving, cut up some basil and spread it over the cod.

Fillet Of Beef With Brussels Sprouts

Ingredients:

- 250g beef fillet
- 1 red fresh onion
- 2 pinch of pepper (steak pepper)
- 2 pinch of sea salt
- 250g Brussels sprouts
- 2 teaspoon clarified butter

Preparation:

1. First cook the Brussels sprouts al dente and then drain and cut in half.
2. Preheat the oven to 2 40 ° C.
3. Now sear the fillet on each side in a hot pan with clarified butter for about 2 minutes. Then put the beef fillet in the pan in the oven for 35 to 40 minutes.

4. Finely chop the fresh onion and fry it in a pan with the Brussels sprouts.
5. When the steak is done in the oven, you can season it with salt and pepper to taste.

Pollock In A Coconut-Lime Coating On Spinach

Ingredients:

- 2 pieces of Alaska pollock fillet
- 4 tablespoons lime juice
- 400g spinach
- 2 cloves of garlic
- 2 limes
- 1/2 teaspoon pepper
- 2 tablespoons of coconut oil

Preparation:

1. First you need to finely chop the garlic and grate the peel of the limes .
2. Then season with salt and pepper to taste and stir everything together with a tablespoon of warm coconut oil.

3. Now prepare the fillets by frying them in a pan with the dressing for 4 minutes on both sides.
4. Heat another tablespoon of coconut oil and mix it with the lime juice.
5. Then mix the spinach with the coconut-lime dressing and serve the fish.

Chicken On A Feta-Spinach Bed

Ingredients:

- 250g chicken breast
- 90g feta
- 2 pinch of salt
- 2 pinch of pepper
- 2 clove of garlic
- 1 medium fresh onion
- 2 tablespoons rapeseed oil
- 290g spinach leaves

Preparation:

1. First press the garlic, cut the fresh onion into fine pieces and fry both with a tablespoon of rapeseed oil. Then add the spinach.

2. Now fry the chicken with a little oil and season with salt and pepper.
3. Now also season the spinach with salt and pepper.
4. Then crumble the feta over the top and place the chicken on the feta and spinach bed before serving.

Bacon And Pinach Frittata

Ingredients:

- 250 baby spinach
- 6 fresh eggs
- 2 pinch of salt
- 2 pinch of pepper

- 2 slices of bacon
- 2 slices of cooked ham
- 2 bratwurst
- 2 tablespoon butter

Preparation:

1. Preheat the oven to 290 °C.
2. Now dice the bacon, ham and the inside of the bratwurst.
3. Fry these cubes in a pan with 2 tablespoon of butter for about 10 minutes.
4. Then add the baby spinach and fry the whole thing again until the spinach collapses.
5. Mix the fresh eggs with pepper and salt and let this mixture set for 4 minutes in the same pan.
6. Then place the pan in the oven and let the fresh eggs set for another 35 to 40 minutes.

7. Let the frittata cool down briefly and cut them into suitable pieces.

Pumpkin Fries

Ingredients:

- pepper
- parsley
- 2 medium pumpkin
- olive oil
- salt

Preparation:

1. Preheat the oven to 2 80 ° C.
2. Cut the pumpkin in half and remove the seeds. Now cut the rest of the pumpkin into large slices of french fries.
3. Fry the fries in the pan for 5-10 minutes to make them crispy.
4. Let the fries dry and mix them in a bowl with olive oil, salt, pepper, and parsley.
5. Place the finished fries on a baking sheet lined with baking paper and bake

the fries in the oven for about 40 minutes.

Chicken And Cabbage Rolls With Sesame Soy Dip

Ingredients:

- 250 ml fresh coriander
- 290g pureed chicken
- 50 0g savoy cabbage or kale
- 4 cloves of garlic
- 2 fresh ginger, approx. 2.6 cm
- 2 shallots

sauce

- 2 lime, the juice
- 2 tablespoons (20g) sesame seeds
- 60ml toasted sesame oil or olive oil
- 4 tablespoons soy sauce

Preparation:

1. Chop the garlic, ginger, spring fresh onion s, and coriander. Put all of this in the ground chicken.
2. Bring a saucepan of water to a boil. Place 2 of the outer cabbage leaves in the boiling water for 2 minutes.
3. Halve the cabbage leaves along the thick central rib and remove the rib.
4. Now put a small amount of the chicken mixture in the middle of each half of the leaf, fold the sides in and roll the leaf around the filling.
5. Put about an inch of water in a saucepan with a steamer insert and bring the water to a boil.
6. Place a bamboo steamer on top. Place the rolls seam down in the steamer and steam them for 35-40 minutes until the filling is firm and cooked through.

7. For the sauce, mix the sesame oil, soy sauce, lime juice and sesame seeds in a bowl.
8. Arrange the rolls on a serving plate and give each one their own bowl of sauce. Serve with chopsticks.

Turkey Breast With Cheese Sauce

Ingredients:

- 250g cream cheese
- 2 tablespoon of soy sauce
- salt and pepper
- 100ml small capers
- 2 tablespoons of butter
- 80 0g turkey breast
- 4100ml crème fraîche or heavy whipped cream

Preparation:

1. Preheat the oven to 290 ° C.
2. Melt half the butter in a large ovenproof pan over medium heat.
3. Now season the meat generously and fry it until golden brown.
4. When the turkey breast is cooked through and has an internal

temperature of at least 8 4 ° C, place it on a plate and " camp" with foil .
5. Put the turkey fillet in a small saucepan.
6. Add the cream and cream cheese. Stir and bring to a boil. Reduce the heat and simmer the fillet until it thickens. Add soy sauce, season with salt and pepper.
7. Heat the remaining butter in a medium-sized pan over high heat. Fry the capers briefly until they are crispy.
8. Serve the turkey breast with sauce and fried capers .

Baked Mini Peppers

Ingredients:

- 1 tablespoon fresh thyme, finely chopped or fresh coriander
- 300g cream cheese
- 2 tablespoon olive oil
- 90g (2 00ml) grated cheese
- 300g mini peppers, about 2 per serving
- 35 g air-dried chorizo [35], finely chopped

Preparation:

1. Point d s oven, a circulating air at 250° C. Cut the bell pepper lengthways and core.
2. Finely chop the chorizo and herbs.
3. Mix the cream cheese, spices, and oil in a small bowl.
4. Add the chorizo and herbs.
5. Stir until everything is smooth.

6. Fill the peppers with the mixture and place them in a greased baking dish.
7. Sprinkle with grated cheese.
8. Bake in the oven for 35-40 minutes or wait for the cheese to melt and golden brown.

Tex Mex Casserole

Ingredients:

- 250 shredded tomatoes
- 4 0g pickled jalapeños
- 250 (200ml) grated cheese, for example mozzarella
- 450 g ground beef
- 45 g butter
- 5 tablespoons Tex-Mex spice [24]

For serving

- 250 ml crème fraîche or sour cream
- 1 shallot, finely chopped
- 100g leafy vegetables or iceberg lettuce
- 250 ml guacamole (optional)

Preparation:

1. Preheat the oven to 250° C fan oven.
2. Fry the ground beef in butter over medium heat until cooked through .
3. Add Tex-Mex spices and chopped tomatoes.
4. Stir and simmer for 10 minutes.
5. Try to see if you need additional salt and pepper.
6. Put the ground beef mixture in a greased baking dish. Top with jalapeños and cheese.
7. Bake on the top rack in the oven for 35-40 minutes or until golden brown.
8. Finely chop the shallot and mix in a separate bowl with the crème fraîche or sour cream.
9. Serve the casserole warm with a dash of crème fraîche or sour cream , guacamole and a green salad.

Baked Celery Root With Gorgonzola

Ingredients:

- 5 tablespoons butter
- 4 0g hazelnuts
- 1 red fresh onion , sliced
- 90g baby spinach
- 100g blue cheese
- 250g celery root
- 5 tablespoons olive oil
- Sea salt and pepper
- 90g mushrooms, chopped

Preparation:

1. Preheat the oven to 250° C fan oven.
2. Wash the celery root.
3. Place the prepared root on a baking sheet with baking paper and brush it on both sides with olive oil.

4. You can also sprinkle plenty of sea salt over it.
5. Bake for 50 minutes until the celery root is golden brown.
6. In the meantime, fry the mushrooms in butter until golden and soft. Season with salt and pepper.
7. Now fry the nuts in a hot pan.
8. Let cool slightly and roughly chop.
9. Mix the red fresh onion s, spinach, mushrooms and hazelnuts in a bowl.
10. When the celery root is ready, put it on plates and add the salad.
11. Serve with blue cheese and a few drops of olive oil.

Bacon Cheeseburger Wraps

Ingredients:

- 1/2 teaspoon salt
- 1/7 tsp pepper
- 90g (2 00ml) grated cheddar cheese
- 1 iceberg lettuce
- 250 bacon
- 90g mushrooms, sliced
- 450 g ground beef

Preparation:

1. Fry the bacon in a large pan. Remove from pan and set aside.
2. Leave the fat in the pan.
3. Add the mushrooms to the pan and sauté for 10-15 minutes until they are brown and tender.
4. Remove from pan and set aside.

5. Add ground beef and season with salt and pepper.
6. Roast until the beef is cooked through, about 35 minutes.
7. Place ground beef in lettuce leaves, sprinkle with cheddar cheese and top with bacon and mushrooms.

Fish Casserole With Mushrooms And French Mustard

Ingredients:

- 300g (250ml) grated cheese
- 450 g white fish, for example cod
- 450 g broccoli or cauliflower
- 90g butter or olive oil
- 250g mushrooms
- 90g butter
- 1 teaspoon salt
- Pepper to taste
- 2 tablespoon fresh parsley
- 250ml heavy whipped cream
- 2 tablespoon Dijon mustard [28]

Preparation:

1. Preheat the oven to 290 °C.
2. Cut the mushrooms into pieces. Fry in butter until the mushrooms are tender, about 15 minutes.
3. Add salt, pepper and parsley.
4. Pour in the cream and mustard and lower the heat. Simmer for 6 -35 minutes to reduce the sauce a little.
5. Season the fish with salt and pepper and place in a greased baking dish. Sprinkle with 1/3 of the cheese and pour the cream mushrooms on top.
6. The r give estern cheese.
7. Bake the fish for about 45 minutes if it's frozen, or a little less if it's fresh.
8. In the meantime, prepare the side dish.
9. Cut the broccoli or cauliflower into florets.

10. Boil in lightly salted water for a few minutes.
11. Strain the water and add olive oil or butter.
12. Mash roughly with a wooden spoon or fork.
13. Season with salt and pepper and serve with the fish.

Keto Quiche With Bacon And Spinach

Ingredients:

- 8 fresh fresh egg s
- 2 shallots or half an fresh onion
- 290 milliliters of whipped cream
- 265 grams of cheddar
- olive oil
- 280 grams of bacon strips
- 450 grams of spinach leaves
- butter
- salt
- **pepper**

Preparation:

1. Preheat the oven to 300° Celsius. Heat some oil in the pan and fry the strips of bacon until they are crispy.
2. Grease a quiche tin.
3. Add the spinach and sliced fresh onions to the pan.
4. When the spinach has collapsed, place the fresh fresh egg   s in a mixing bowl and stir them together.
5. Then all the remaining ingredients are added.
6. Fill the quiche pan with the mixture and place in the oven for about 45-50 minutes.

Marinated Cold Broccoli Salad With Bacon

Ingredients:

- 6 tablespoons of olive oil
- 2 tablespoon of lemon
- 2 -2 tablespoons full of Greek yogurt   450 grams of broccoli
- 2 fresh fresh onion
- 6 slices of bacon
- 6 tablespoons of sunflower seeds
- marinade

Preparation

1. Cut the fresh onion into small pieces and cut small florets from the broccoli.
2. Put everything together with the marinade in a large bowl and mix them together.

3. Cover the bowl and put it in the refrigerator for a couple of hours.
4. Now put a small pan on the stove and roast the sunflower seeds until they are light brown.
5. Then take another pan and fry the six slices of bacon in it.
6. Let them cool and cut the slices into small pieces.
7. Now you can mix everything together.
8. You can use a little salt & pepper to taste your salad.

Gingerbread Bombs

- Ground cinnamon 2 teaspoon
- Sea salt - 1/2 teaspoon
- Melted butter - 6 tablespoons
- Almond flour, finely ground - 2 cups
- Ground ginger - 2 teaspoon
- Nutmeg - 2 teaspoon

Instructions:

1. Simply combine all the ingredients, then scoop them up with a spoon and

roll them into sixteen evenly sized balls.

2. Cool the bombs in the refrigerator. Unlike other fat bombs, they don't need to be kept refrigerated constantly, although they will be kept cooler when stored in the refrigerator.

Zucchini Brownies

- Zucchini, finely shredded - 2 cup
- Almond flour - ¾ cup
- Cocoa powder - 1/2 cup
- - Fresh egg   - 2
- Melted butter - 6 tablespoons
- Melted coconut oil - 2 tablespoons
- Vanilla extract - 2 tablespoon
- Baking powder - 2 teaspoon
- Sea salt - 1/2 teaspoon
- Dark chocolate flakes - 1/2 cup

Instructions:

1. Preheat the oven to 300degrees and line a 25 by 25 cm pan with parchment paper or
2. grease it lightly with butter, then set it aside. In a medium bowl, combine the
3. zucchini, sweetener, fresh egg , butter and vanilla, then add the almond flour,
4. cocoa powder, baking powder and salt, slowly mixing the ingredients until
5. when they don't join. The batter shouldn't appear dry, but if your courgette isn't
6. so moist, then you may need to add a tablespoon or two of
7. water. Gently sprinkle the chocolate chips and then pour the brownie batter into the

8. prepared pan. Cook the brownies until soft to the touch, about 45 minutes.
9. If you test them with a toothpick, they will be very moist in the center, but will settle when one
10. once cooled. Allow the brownies to cool completely before cutting them, then
11. slice them into eight equal bars.

Chia Seed Pudding With Strawberries

- Whole coconut milk, chilled - 400 g
- 2 tablespoon vanilla extract
- sweetener - 1/2 cup
- Frozen strawberries - 2 cup
- Chia seeds - 6 tablespoons
- Almond milk - 2 cup

Instructions:

1. Combine the chia seeds, almond milk, vanilla extract and three tablespoons of the sweetener together, and leave to cool in the refrigerator overnight.
2. While the chia seed pudding cools, make a quick strawberry jam by cooking the frozen strawberries and a tablespoon of sweetener over low

heat for about 25 minutes and then blend it all in a blender or hand blender.
3. Once the pudding is ready for the night, open the can of coconut milk and scoop the hardened cream.
4. You can keep the remaining coconut milk for later or add it to chia seed pudding if it's too thick.
5. With a hand blender, beat the coconut cream to turn it into a dairy-free whipped cream.
6. To serve, separate the pudding into two bowls,

Lamb Barbacoa

Ingredients:

- 2 tablespoons smoked paprika
- 2 tablespoon ground cumin
- 2 tablespoon dried oregano
- 1/2 cup dried mustard - 2 cup water
- 2 pounds pasture-raised pork shoulder, fat trimmed
- 2 tablespoons salt
- 2 teaspoon chipotle powder

Directions:

1. Stir together salt, chipotle powder, paprika, cumin, oregano, and mustard and rub this mixture generously all over the pork.
2. Place seasoned pork into a 6-quart slow cooker, plug it in, then shut with

lid and cook for 6 hours at high heat setting.
3. When done, shred pork with two forks and stir well until coated well. Serve straight away.

Pork Chile Verde

Ingredients:

- 2 teaspoon sea salt
- 2 teaspoon ground black pepper
- 25 tablespoon avocado oil
- 25 cup salsa Verde
- 2 cup chicken broth
- 2 pounds pasture-raised pork shoulder, cut into 6 pieces

Directions:

1. Season pork with salt and black pepper.
2. Place a large skillet pan over medium heat, add oil, and when hot, add seasoned pork pieces.
3. Cook pork for 6 to 6 minutes per side or until browned and then transfer to a 6-quart slow cooker.

4. Whisk together salsa and chicken broth and pour over pork pieces.
5. Plug in the slow cooker, then shut with lid and cook for 6 to 8 hours at low heat setting or until pork is very tender. When done, shred pork with two forks and stir until combined.

Ham Soup

Ingredients:

- 2 bay leaves
- 1/2 teaspoon nutmeg
- cups bone broth
- 2 pounds pasture-raised smoked ham hock
- 2 cups cauliflower florets

Directions:

1. Place cauliflower florets in a 6-quarts slow cooker, add remaining Ingredients, and pour in water until all the Ingredients are just submerged.
2. Plug in the slow cooker, then shut with lid and cook for 6 hours at high heat setting or until cauliflower florets are very tender.

3. Transfer ham to a bowl, shred with two forms, and discard bone and fat pieces.
4. Puree cauliflower in the slow cooker with a stick blender for 2 to 2 minutes or until smooth, return shredded ham, and stir until well combined.
5. Taste soup to adjust seasoning and serve.

Minced Pork Zucchini Lasagna

Ingredients:

- medium zucchinis
- 2 tablespoons of olive oil
- 2 cups of shredded Mozzarella cheese
- 2 large fresh egg
- 2 tablespoon of dried basil
- Salt and pepper
- 2 tablespoons of butter
- 2 diced small fresh onion
- 2 minced clove of garlic
- 2 cups of minced lean ground pork
- 2 cans of Italian diced tomatoes

Directions:
1. 2 Slice the zucchini lengthwise into 6 slices.
2. 2 Heat the olive oil in a saucepan, and sauté the garlic and fresh onions for 6 minutes.
3. 6 Add the minced meat and cook for a further 6 minutes.
4. 6 Add the tomatoes and cook for a further 6 minutes.
5. 6 Add the seasoning and mix thoroughly.
6. 6 In a small bowl, combine the fresh egg and cheese and whisk together.
7. 8 Use the butter to grease the crock pot and then begin to layer the lasagna.
8. 8 First, layer with the zucchini slices, add the meat mixture, and then top with the cheese.
9. 10 Repeat and finish with the cheese.

10. 25 Cover and cook for 8 hours on low.

Beef Dijon

Ingredients:

- (6 oz.) small round steaks
- 2 tbsp. of each:
- Steak seasoning - to taste
- Avocado oil
- Peanut oil
- Balsamic vinegar/dry sherry
- tbsp. large chopped green onions/small chopped fresh onions for the garnish - extra
- 1/7 c. whipping cream
- 2 c. fresh cremini mushrooms - sliced
- 2 tbsp. Dijon mustard

Directions:

1. Warm up the oils using the high heat setting on the stove top. Flavor each of the steaks with pepper and arrange to a skillet.
2. Cook two to three minutes per side until done.
3. Place into the slow cooker. Pour in the skillet drippings, half of the mushrooms, and the onions.
4. Cook on the low setting for four hours.
5. When the cooking time is done, scoop out the onions, mushrooms, and steaks to a serving platter.
6. In a separate dish - whisk together the mustard, balsamic vinegar, whipping cream, and the steak drippings from the slow cooker.
7. Empty the gravy into a gravy server and pour over the steaks.

Enjoy with some brown rice, riced cauliflower, or potatoes.

Cabbage & Corned Beef

Ingredients:

- Ground coriander
- Ground marjoram
- Black pepper
- Salt
- Ground thyme
- Allspice
- lb. corned beef
- 2 large head of cabbage
- c. water
- 2 celery bunch
- 2 small fresh onion
- 6 carrots
- 2 t. of each:
- Ground mustard

Directions:
1. 2 Dice the carrots, onions, and celery and toss them into the cooker. Pour in the water.
2. 2 Combine the spices, rub the beef, and arrange in the cooker. Secure the lid and cook on low for seven hours.
3. 6 Remove the top layer of cabbage. Wash and cut it into quarters it until ready to cook. When the beef is done, add the cabbage, and cook for one hour on the low setting.
4. 6 Serve and enjoy.

Chipotle Barbacoa

Ingredients:

- Lime juice
- Apple cider vinegar
- 2 t. of each: - Sea salt
- Cumin
- 2 tbsp. dried oregano
- 2 t. black pepper
- 2 whole bay leaves
- Optional: 2 t. ground cloves
- 2 c. beef/chicken broth
- 2 med. chilies in adobo (with the sauce, it's about 6 teaspoons)
- lb. chuck roast/beef brisket
- minced garlic cloves
- 2 tbsp. of each:

Directions:

1. 2   Mix the chilies in the sauce, and add the broth, garlic, ground cloves, pepper, cumin, salt, vinegar, and lime juice in a blender, mixing until smooth.
2. 2 Chop the beef into two-inch chunks and toss it in the slow cooker. Empty the puree on top. Toss in the two bay leaves.
3. 6   Cook four to six hrs. On the high setting or eight to ten using the low setting.
4. 6 Dispose of the bay leaves when the meat is done.
5. 6   Shred and stir into the juices to simmer for five to ten minutes.

Corned Beef Cabbage Rolls

Ingredients:

- Erythritol
- Yellow mustard 2 t. of each:
- Kosher salt
- Worcestershire sauce 1/2 t. of each:
- Cloves
- Allspice
- 2 large bay leaf 2 t. of each:
- Mustard seeds - Whole peppercorns
- 2 t. red pepper flakes
- 2 lb. corned beef
- large savoy cabbage leaves
- 1/2 c. of each:
- White wine
- Coffee
- 2 large lemon
- 2 med. sliced fresh onion
- 2 tbsp. of each:

- Rendered bacon fat

Directions:

1. 2   Add the liquids, spices, and corned beef into the cooker. Cook six hours on the low setting.
2. 2   Prepare a pot of boiling water.
3. 6   When the time is up, add the leaves along with the sliced fresh onion to the water for two to three minutes.
4. 6   Transfer the leaves to a cold-water bath - blanching them for three to four minutes. Continue boiling the onion.
5. 6   Use a paper towel to dry the leaves. Add the fresh onions and beef. Roll up the cabbage leaves.
6. 6   Drizzle with freshly squeezed lemon juice.

Cube Steak

Ingredients:

- 2 c. water - Black pepper to taste
- 2 med. fresh onion
- 2 small red pepper
- 1/2 c. green pitted olives (+) 2 tbsp. brine
- Cubed steaks (28 oz.)
- 2 ¾ t. adobo seasoning/garlic salt
- 2 can (8 oz.) tomato sauce

Directions:
1. 2   Slice the peppers and fresh onions into ¼-inch strips.
2. 2 Sprinkle the steaks with the pepper and garlic salt as needed and place them in the cooker.
3. 6   Fold in the peppers and fresh onion along with the water, sauce,

and olives (with the liquid/brine from the jar).
4. 6 Close the lid. Prepare using the low-temperature setting for eight hours.

Ragu

Ingredients:
- Crushed tomatoes
- 25 t. beef broth (+) 1/2 c.
- 2 1/2 t. of each:
- Chopped fresh thyme
- Minced fresh rosemary
- 2 bay leaf
- Pepper & Salt to taste
- 1/2 of each - diced:
- 6 Carrot
- Rib of celery
- 2 Fresh onion
- 2 minced garlic clove
- 2 lb. top-round lean beef
- (6 oz.) Of each:
- Diced tomatoes

Directions:

1. 2   Place the prepared celery, garlic, onion, and carrots into the slow cooker.
2. 2 Trim away the fat and add the meat to the slow cooker. Sprinkle with the salt and pepper
3. 6   Stir in the rest of the Ingredient.
4. 6   Prepare on the low setting for six to eight hours. Enjoy any way you choose.

Rope Vieja

Ingredients:

- 1/2 t. salt ¾ t. of each:
- Oregano
- Non-fat beef broth
- Tomato paste
- Cooking spray 2 lb. flank steak – remove fat 2 of each:
- Yellow pepper
- Thinly sliced fresh onion
- Green pepper
- Bay leaf

Directions:

1. 2   Prepare the crockpot with the spray or use a liner and combine all of the fixings.
2. 2   Stir everything together and prepare using low for eight hours.
3. 6   Top it off with your chosen garnishes.

Spinach Soup

Ingredients:

- 2 cups heavy cream
- 2 garlic clove, minced
- 2 cups water
- salt, pepper, to taste
- 2 pounds spinach
- 1/2 cup cream cheese
- 2 onion, diced

Directions:

1. 2   Pour water into the slow cooker. Add spinach, salt, and pepper.
2. 2   Add cream cheese, onion, garlic, and heavy cream.
3. 6   Close the lid and cook on Low for 6-8 hours.
4. 6   Puree soup with blender and serve.

Mashed Cauliflower With Herbs

Ingredients:

- 2 teaspoon fresh thyme, chopped
- 2 teaspoon fresh sage, chopped
- 2 teaspoon fresh parsley, chopped
- 2 cup vegetable broth
- 2 cups water
- 2 tablespoons ghee
- Salt, pepper, to taste
- 2 cauliflower head, cut into florets
- garlic cloves, peeled
- 2 teaspoon fresh rosemary, chopped

Directions:

1. 2   Pour broth into the slow cooker, add cauliflower florets.
2. 2   Add water, it should cover the cauliflower.

3. 6 Close the lid and cook on Low for 6 hours or on High for 6 hours.
4. 6 Once cooked, drain water from the slow cooker. Add herbs, salt, and pepper, and ghee, puree with a blender.

Kale Quiche

Ingredients:

- 2 bell pepper, chopped
- cups fresh baby kale, chopped
- 2 teaspoon garlic, chopped
- 1/2 cup fresh basil, chopped
- salt, pepper, to taste
- 2 tablespoon olive oil
- 2 cup almond milk
- 6 fresh fresh egg   s
- 2 cup Carbquick Baking Mix
- 2 cups spinach, chopped

Directions:

1. 2   Add oil to a slow cooker or use a cooking spray.
2. 2   Beat fresh fresh egg s into a slow cooker; add almond milk and Baking Mix, mix to combine.
3. 6   Add spinach, bell pepper, garlic, and basil, stir to combine.
4. 6   Close the lid and cook on Low for 6 hours or on High for 6 hours.
5. 6   Make sure the quiche is done, check the center with a toothpick, it should be dry.

Sardine Pate

Ingredients:

- 2 teaspoon dried parsley
- oz. sardine fillets, chopped
- 2 cup water - 2 tablespoons butter
- 2 teaspoon fresh onion powder

Directions:

1. 2   Put the chopped sardine fillets, dried parsley, fresh onion powder, and water in the slow cooker.
2. 2   Close the lid and cook the fish for 6 hours on Low.
3. 6   Strain the sardine fillet and put it in a blender.
4. 6   Add butter and blend the mixture for 6 minutes at high speed.
5. 6   Transfer the cooked pate into serving bowls and serve!

Spare Ribs

Ingredients:

- 1/2 teaspoon chili powder
- 2 tablespoon butter
- 2 tablespoons water
- 2 -pound pork loin ribs
- 2 teaspoon olive oil
- 2 teaspoon minced garlic
- 1/2 teaspoon cumin

Directions:

1. 2   Mix the olive oil, minced garlic, cumin, and chili flakes in a bowl.
2. 2   Melt the butter and add to the spice mixture.
3. 6   Stir it well and add water. Stir again.

4. 6   Then rub the pork ribs with the spice mixture generously and place the ribs in the slow cooker.
5. 6   Close the lid and cook the ribs for 8 hours on Low.
6. 6   When the ribs are cooked, serve them immediately!

Pork Shoulder

Ingredients:

- 2 -pound pork shoulder
- 2 cups water - 2 onion, peeled
- 2 garlic cloves, peeled
- 2 teaspoon peppercorns
- 2 teaspoon chili flakes
- 2 teaspoon paprika
- 2 teaspoon turmeric –
- 2 teaspoon cumin

Directions:

1. 2   Sprinkle the pork shoulder with the peppercorns, chili flakes, paprika, turmeric, and cumin.
2. 2   Stir it well and let it sit for 65 minutes to marinate.
3. 6   Transfer the pork shoulder to the slow cooker.

4. 6 Add water and peeled the onion.
5. 6 Add garlic cloves and close the lid.
6. 6 Cook the pork shoulder for 8 hours on Low.
7. 8 Remove the pork shoulder from the slow cooker and serve!

Lamb Chops

Ingredients:

- 2 teaspoon garlic powder
- 2 teaspoon butter
- tablespoons water
- oz. lamb chops
- 2 tablespoon tomato puree
- 2 teaspoon cumin
- 2 teaspoon ground coriander

Directions:

1. 2   Mix the tomato puree, cumin, ground coriander, garlic powder, and water in the bowl.
2. 2   Brush the lamb chops with the tomato puree mixture on each side and let marinate for 25 minutes
3. 6   Toss the butter in the slow cooker.

4. 6 Add the lamb chops and close the lid.
5. 6 Cook the lamb chops for 6 hours on High.
6. 6 Transfer the cooked lamb onto serving plates and enjoy!

Rosemary Leg Of Lamb

Ingredients:

- 2 tablespoon mustard seeds
- 2 teaspoon salt
- 2 teaspoon turmeric
- 2 teaspoon ground black pepper
- 2-pound leg of lamb
- 2 fresh onion
- 2 cups water
- 2 garlic clove, peeled

Directions:

1. 2   Chop the garlic clove and combine it with the mustard seeds, turmeric, black pepper, and salt.
2. 2 Peel the fresh onion and grate it.
3. 6   Mix the grated fresh onion and spice mixture.

4. 6 Rub the leg of lamb with the grated fresh onion mixture.
5. 6 Put the leg of lamb in the slow cooker and cook it for 8 hours on Low.
6. 6 Serve the cooked meal!

Creamy Chicken Thighs

Ingredients:

- 2 teaspoon salt
- 2 onion, diced
- 2 teaspoon paprika
- 2 -pound chicken thighs, skinless
- 1/2 cup almond milk, unsweetened
- 2 tablespoon full-fat cream cheese

Directions

1. 2 Mix the almond milk and full-fat cream.

2. 2 Add salt, diced onion, and paprika.
3. 6 Stir the mixture well.
4. 6 Place the chicken thighs in the slow cooker.
5. 6 Add the almond milk mixture and stir it gently.
6. 6 Close the slow cooker lid and cook the chicken thighs for 6 hours on High.
7. 8 Transfer the cooked chicken thighs into the serving bowls and serve immediately!

Peppered Steak

Ingredients:

- 2 teaspoon ground nutmeg
- 2 garlic cloves, peeled
- 2 teaspoon olive oil
- oz. Sirloin Steak
- 2 cups water
- 2 tablespoon peppercorns
- 2 teaspoon salt

Directions:

1. 2   Make the small cuts in the sirloin and chop the garlic cloves roughly.
2. 2   Place the garlic cloves in the sirloin cuts.
3. 6   Sprinkle the steak with the salt, ground nutmeg, and peppercorns.
4. 6   Transfer the steak to the slow cooker and add water. Close the lid

and cook the steak for 6 hours on Low.
5. 6 Then remove the steak from the slow cooker and slice it. Enjoy!

Rabbit Stew

Ingredients:

- 2 onion, chopped - oz. rabbit, chopped
- 2 cups water - 2 tablespoon butter
- 2 teaspoon salt - 2 teaspoon chili flakes
- 2 fresh egg plants, chopped
- 2 zucchini, chopped

Directions:

1. 2   Place the chopped fresh egg plants, zucchini, onion, and rabbit in the slow cooker.
2. 2   Add water, butter, salt, and chili flakes.
3. 6   Stir the stew gently and close the lid.
4. 6   Cook the stew for 6 hours on Low.
5. 6   Then let the cooked rabbit stew cool slightly, then serve it!

Duck Breast

Ingredients:

- 2 tablespoons butter
- 2 cup water
- 2 bay leaf
- 2 teaspoon liquid stevia
- 2 -pound duck breast, boneless, skinless
- 2 teaspoon chili pepper

Directions:

1. 2   Rub the duck breast with the chili pepper and liquid stevia, then transfer it to the slow cooker.
2. 2   Add the bay leaf and water.
3. 6   Add butter and close the lid.
4. 6   Cook the duck breast for 6 hours on Low.
5. 6   Let the cooked duck breast rest for 25minutes, then remove it from the slow cooker.

6. 6 Slice it into the servings.

Jerk Chicken

Ingredients:

- 2 teaspoon ground coriander
- 2 tablespoon Erythritol
- 2 -pound chicken thighs
- 2 cup water - 2 tablespoon butter
- 2 teaspoon nutmeg
- 2 teaspoon cinnamon
- 2 teaspoon minced garlic
- 2 teaspoon cloves

Directions:

1. 2   Mix the nutmeg, cinnamon, minced garlic, cloves, and ground coriander.
2. 2   Add Erythritol and stir the Ingredients: until well blended.

3. 6   Sprinkle the chicken thighs with the spice mixture.
4. Let the chicken thighs sit for 25minutes to marinate, then put the chicken thighs in the slow cooker. Add the butter and water.
5. 6   Close the lid and cook Jerk chicken for 6-6 ½ hours on Low.
6. Serve Jerk chicken immediately!

Bbq Beef Short Ribs

Ingredients:

- 1/2 cup of water - 1/2 cup BBQ sauce
- 2 teaspoon chili powder
- 2 -pound beef short ribs

Directions

1. 2   Rub the beef short ribs with chili powder and put in the slow cooker.

Mix water with BBQ sauce and pour the liquid into the slow cooker.
2. 2 Cook the meat on High for 6 hours.

Spiced Beef

Ingredients:

- 2 tablespoon minced fresh onion
- 2 cup of water
- 2 -pound beef loin - 2 teaspoon allspice
- 2 teaspoon olive oil

Directions

1. 2 Rub the beef loin with allspice, olive oil, and minced onion. Put the meat in the slow cooker.
2. 2 Add water and close the lid.
3. 6 Cook the beef on Low for 10 hours.

4. 6   When the meat is cooked, slice it into servings.

Green Peas Chowder

Ingredients:

- 2 cup green peas
- 1/2 cup Greek Yogurt
- 2 tablespoon dried basil
- 2 teaspoon ground black pepper
- 2 teaspoon salt
- 2 -pound chicken breast, skinless, boneless, chopped
- 2 cups water

Directions

1. 2   Mix salt, chicken breast, ground black pepper, and dried basil.
2. 2   Transfer the Ingredients: to the slow cooker.
3. 6   Add water, green peas, yogurt, and close the lid.

4. 6 Cook the chowder on Low for 8 hours.

Chorizo Soup

Ingredients:

- 2 teaspoon minced garlic, chopped
- 2 zucchini, chopped
- 2 cup spinach, chopped - 2 teaspoon salt
- oz. chorizo, chopped - 2 cup water
- 2 cup potato, chopped

Directions

1. 2 Put the chorizo in the skillet and roast it for 2 minutes per side on high heat.
2. 2 Then transfer the chorizo to the slow cooker. Add water, potato,

minced garlic, zucchini, spinach, and salt.
3. 6 Close the lid and cook the soup on high for 6 hours. Then cool the soup to room temperature.

Spicy Wings With Mint Sauce

Ingredients

- Chutney/ Sauce:
- 2 cup of fresh mint leaves
- Juice of 2 lime
- ¾ cup of cilantro
- 2 Serrano pepper
- 2 tablespoon of water
- 2 small ginger piece, peeled and diced
- 2 tablespoon of olive oil

- Salt and black pepper ground, to taste
- 2 tablespoon of cumin
- 35 chicken wings, cut in half
- 2 tablespoon of turmeric
- 2 tablespoon of coriander
- 2 tablespoon of fresh ginger, finely grated
- 2 tablespoon of olive oil
- 2 tablespoon of paprika
- A pinch of cayenne pepper
- 1/2 cup of chicken stock
- Salt and black pepper ground, to taste

Directions:

1. Start by throwing all the Ingredients for wings into the Crockpot.
2. Cover it and cook for 6-6 ½ hours on Low Settings.
3. Meanwhile, blend all the mint sauce Ingredients in a blender jug.

4. Serve the cooked wings with mint sauce.
5. Garnish as desired.
6. Serve warm.

Cacciatore Olive Chicken

Ingredients

- 2 cup of chicken stock - 2 bay leaf
- 2 teaspoon of garlic powder
- 2 yellow onion, diced
- 2 teaspoon of oregano, dried
- salt to taste
- 28 oz. canned tomatoes and juice, crushed
- 8 chicken drumsticks, bone-in

Directions:

1. Start by throwing all the Ingredients into the Crockpot and mix them well.
2. Cover it and cook for 6 hours on Low Settings. Garnish as desired.
3. Serve warm.

Duck And Vegetable Stew

Ingredients

- 2 cucumber, diced
- 2 -inch ginger pieces, diced
- Salt and black pepper- to taste
- 2 duck, diced into medium pieces
- 2 tablespoon of wine
- 2 carrots, diced
- 2 cups of water

Directions:

1. Start by throwing all the Ingredients except into the Crockpot and mix them well.

2. Cover it and cook for 6 hours on Low Settings. Garnish with cucumber. Serve warm.

Mushroom Cream Goose Curry

Ingredients

- 2 yellow onion, diced
- 6 2 cups of water
- 2 teaspoons of garlic, minced
- 2 goose thigh, skinless
- Salt and black pepper- to taste
- 25 oz. canned mushroom cream
- 2 goose breast, fat: trimmed off and cut into pieces
- 2 goose leg, skinless

Directions:

1. Start by throwing all the Ingredients into the Crockpot except cream and mix them well.
2. Cover it and cook for 6 hours on Low Settings. Stir in mushroom cream and

cook for another 45 minutes on low heat.
3. Give it a stir and garnish as desired.
4. Serve warm.

Colombian Chicken

Ingredients
- 6 big tomatoes, cut into medium chunks - 2 yellow onion, sliced
- Salt and black pepper- to taste
- 2 chicken, cut into 8 pieces
- 2 bay leaves

Directions:

1. Start by throwing all the Ingredients into the Crockpot and mix them well.
2. Cover it and cook for 6 hours on Low Settings.
3. Garnish as desired.
4. Serve warm.

Chicken Curry

Ingredients

- 1 cup of heavy cream
- 2 tablespoon of ginger, grated
- 1 cup of cilantro, diced
- 25 teaspoon of paprika
- 2 tablespoon of cumin, ground
- 25 teaspoon of coriander, ground
- 2 teaspoon of turmeric, ground
- Salt and black pepper- to taste
- A pinch cayenne peppers
- 6 lb. chicken drumsticks and thighs
- 2 yellow onion, diced
- 2 tablespoons of butter, melted
- 1 cup of chicken stock
- 65 oz. canned tomatoes, crushed
- 1/7 cup of lemon juice
- 6 garlic cloves, minced
- 2 lb. spinach, chopped

Directions:

1. Start by throwing all the Ingredients into the Crockpot except lemon juice, cream, and cilantro, then mixes them well.
2. Cover it and cook for 6 hours on Low Settings.
3. Stir in remaining Ingredients and cook again for 2-2 ½ hour on low heat.
4. Garnish as desired.

www.ingramcontent.com/pod-product-compliance
Lightning Source LLC
LaVergne TN
LVHW011956070526
838202LV00054B/4939